I0053925

BRAIN
INJURY
A PATIENT'S PERSPECTIVE

BY: FRANK AWUKU AMPONSAH

Copyright © 2025 by
Frank Awuku Amponsah

ALL RIGHTS RESERVED.

NO part of this book may be reproduced or transmitted in any form by any means, electronic or mechanical, including photocopying and recording, or by any information storage and retrieval system, except as may be expressly permitted in writing from the author.

Paperback ISBN: 978-1-965875-23-0

Dedication

I would like to dedicate this book to my family for the help and support they provided me in several different ways.

Preface

This is a true account of the experience of a stroke patient to highlight their experience of the NHS in three separate hospitals in London. The hospitals are in completely different geographical areas in different boroughs, although all three are under the NHS trust.

The author has respected GDPR and privacy laws and, as a result, has neither disclosed the names of any of the hospitals nor any names of medical and/or healthcare professionals. Still, every other detail is true and not fictitious. In that respect, the author has given the account of their experience exactly as it is, so some hospitals have the credit they are due. Still, unfortunately, one or more hospitals have a pretty damning description of their care provision. It must be mentioned that it is just the way things are, or rather the way things turned out to be and very much as experienced by the writer. It remains my hope that other brain injury survivors and their families can benefit from reading this book and may be able to use my experience to enrich their personal experience; healthcare professionals may also benefit from reading this book because of the insight it can provide them to see things from the viewpoint of patients in their care.

Table of Contents

CHAPTER 1
HOW IT BEGAN

It all began on a December evening in 2021 when I returned home after riding my bike in our neighbourhood, something I do regularly. That night was different—I was recovering from a cold, so I took it easy. Still, I felt unusually tired and weak on my way back. Instead of reaching for my keys when I arrived at the front door, I simply knocked. My daughter opened the door, took one look at me, and screamed, calling out to my wife, "Mom, I think we need to call an ambulance for Dad! He looks like he's having a stroke".

I overheard her speaking with the paramedics on the phone. It all seemed to be happening so fast. A part of me thought they were overreacting, but I was also confused and unsure of what was happening. I instinctively tried to climb the stairs to my bedroom, wanting to lie down, but I struggled. With my wife's help, I eventually made it there and lay down flat on the floor.

Minutes later, the ambulance crew arrived. I was still in shock as they questioned my wife about what had happened. After she explained, they turned to me for my account of the evening. They checked my blood sugar and blood pressure before carefully helping me into a wheelchair and carrying me downstairs to the waiting ambulance. One of them mentioned they would "blue light" me to Hospital One.

The journey was quick, but it was a dark and damp winter evening. As I lay there, I tried to make out where we were whenever I caught a glimpse through the ambulance window. All I could see were the blurred lights of tall buildings, a sign that we were heading into London. The paramedics were incredibly kind and reassuring throughout the ride, which helped ease my nerves.

ADMISSION TO HOSPITAL ONE

We arrived at the hospital soon, and I was transferred from the ambulance into what looked like the accident and emergency department of a bustling hospital. I remember the doctor telling my wife that I had a blood clot on the right side of my brain and that they wanted my consent to carry out a procedure. I begged him to consider any alternative therapy other than the procedure, if at all possible. Thankfully, he answered in the affirmative but added that he would first need to conduct an MRI scan. I agreed wholeheartedly because, under the circumstances, anything other than surgery was preferable. At that moment, the only thing I knew about strokes was that they typically affected older people. I never realized that a stroke was a type of brain injury, nor did I consider that it might require a surgical procedure to treat. On top of that, there was simply too much happening for me to fully grasp the situation. That confusion led to a state of self-denial, something that lingered even after the stroke. However, as I began researching the illness, my understanding broadened, helping me manage the condition much better.

I was eventually placed on a trolley, though there was an initial delay in getting one. The only available trolley had been used by a patient with COVID-19 symptoms, so it had to be thoroughly wiped down before I could use it. Once it was cleaned, I was placed on it and wheeled into what looked like a giant washing machine—similar to the ones found in a laundry. I closed my eyes, as it was dark inside the machine anyway, and I was pushed further inside along with the trolley. Luckily, the scan was completed within minutes. Still, the medical professionals determined that I needed to remain in the hospital for observation, and eventually, I was admitted to the intensive care unit. The consultant later informed me that the brain scan had revealed a massive stroke and that the quick decision to call an ambulance had been key to my survival. At that moment, the reality of the situation fully sank in. I have to admit—I was scared and overwhelmed by the speed at which everything had unfolded.

I spent Christmas in Hospital One, though it passed so quickly that I barely had time to reflect on it. Frequent visits from my family made my hospital stay much more pleasant than it otherwise would have been, and in some ways, it even felt like being at home, surrounded by my loved ones. Each bed in the ward had a screen displaying the patient's blood pressure, heart rate, and other vital statistics. I spent most of my days in that unit watching that screen.

I remained in bed for the majority of each day because I was extremely weak. Additionally, the healthcare professionals advised me that staying in bed was the safest option, so I had little choice. My treatment began immediately, with nurses visiting the ward twice daily to administer medication to all the patients. I was prescribed about four different medications, all in the form of tablets or capsules, which I took after meals.

In addition to my tablets and capsules, I received an injection approximately every other day. I used to offer my left arm to the nurses because it was so numb that I could barely feel the needle. However, as the numbness gradually faded, I started to feel the pain. Eventually, it didn't matter which arm I used—I would feel that short, sharp sting regardless. Still, the fact that I could feel the injections again was a good sign.

Since I was required to stay in bed, the nurses provided me with a small device to keep by my bedside. I was told to press a button on it whenever I needed help with anything.

CHAPTER 2
TRANSFER TO HOSPITAL TWO

My consultant told me that I would be transferred to a hospital closer to my residence, which I have referred to as Hospital Two. Curious about the reason for the transfer, I inquired and was told that it was because I would be preparing for rehabilitation—the next phase of my recovery process. While the prospect of rehabilitation was encouraging, as it signified that I was on the mend, I couldn't shake my disappointment. Hospital Two had received a lot of bad press, and I was genuinely reluctant about being sent there. Still, I thanked God for my progress and reasoned from my Christian perspective that if it was God's will for me to go to that hospital, then it must be the best place for me.

About two weeks after that conversation, I was once again transferred into an ambulance. This journey was even better than the previous one because it was during the day, and this time, I was fully aware of what was happening and where we were headed. The ambulance crew was fantastic—perhaps even better than the last team—because they were cracking jokes along the way. Since there was no emergency this time, their light-heartedness put me at ease. Their ability to find joy in their work made me feel safe and reassured.

We arrived at Hospital Two well before dark, and I was taken directly to the acute stroke unit. As soon as I arrived at the ward, I was assigned a bed, and the lead consultant, along with two therapists, came to introduce themselves. One of them identified herself as my occupational therapist. I quickly noticed that this ward had significantly more patients than the one I had been in at

Hospital One. However, the patients here seemed to be in different stages of recovery. While most remained in bed, about three or four were walking around the ward with the aid of walking sticks or frames, spending much less time in bed than the others.

My consultant was friendly and introduced me to several ward nurses. Beside my bed, there was a highchair, and the therapists told me that if I wanted to come out of bed, I should ask for assistance to sit in it. Feeling the need to rest, I got into bed with help from my occupational therapist and noticed a television mounted on the ceiling. From my position in bed, I had a clear view of the screen. The nurses informed me that remote control was available, so if I wanted to switch channels from the default NHSTV, I could request it. However, I found NHSTV quite informative and relevant, so I watched it most of the time and even began to enjoy it. Every morning, the nurses would come to wipe me down with a towel and warm water. Later, my occupational therapist returned to my bedside and pinned a piece of information on the noticeboard behind my bed. It displayed details about me, including my name, dietary requirements, consultant's name, and caseworker. She also brought a wheelchair, explaining that it belonged to the ward and that I could use it whenever needed by simply informing the nurses. I soon settled in and started making friends—not just with the nurses and therapists, but also with other patients. The doctors often sat on my bed, engaging in casual conversations and asking whether I felt any new pain.

Unfortunately, I began receiving some hostility from certain nurses. It all started when the lead consultant asked me about my experience in the hospital, and I openly shared my thoughts. One of my concerns was that the nurses frequently disappeared from the ward at times when patients clearly needed assistance with basic care—such as changing the nappies of bedbound patients. In response, one of the nurses bluntly told me that many patients were misdiagnosed under the NHS because they displayed attitudes like mine.

I later found out that this nurse was actually the deputy ward manager. My friction with him escalated one morning when I asked for assistance in repositioning myself in bed, and he outright refused. Frustrated, I pointed out that such behaviour could be considered wilful neglect and, in a corporate business environment, would be grounds for gross misconduct. He walked away but returned later, suspiciously asking whether I was truly a stroke patient or an NHS investigator. He mentioned that he had to attend to an urgent matter downstairs but was still questioning who I really was.

One morning, while struggling to reposition myself in bed, I saw a man walking past and called out to him for help. I pleaded with him to assist me, as I had been lying on my weak side for too long. Instead of helping, he yelled, "Who is going to touch you? And then, when you fall, they will get the blame!" Bewildered, I asked how I could possibly fall while lying in bed. I pointed to the notice behind my bed, written by my consultant, stating that I required help repositioning myself regularly. He simply shrugged and walked away. After that, I learned he had started spreading rumours among the staff that I was a fall risk due to my condition.

The next day, my occupational therapist visited my bedside, and I asked for help sitting in my highchair. She assisted me, and I remained seated for quite a while. When she returned to check on me, I told her I wanted to continue sitting up for a bit longer. She praised my effort, and I explained that I wanted to do activities like this more frequently. She encouraged me to call the nurses if I ever wanted to sit in the chair, but I remarked that they always seemed too busy—when they were even present in the ward.

I then asked when I would have the opportunity to start walking with a stick, like some of the other patients. She assured me she would look into it. Meanwhile, one of the nurses came by to take lunch orders. After selecting my meal, I asked if I could eat in my chair instead of in bed. She said that would be fine but that she would need to bring me a table. When she returned with the table, set my food tray on it, and handed me a new eating jar, I was overjoyed. That day, for the first time since my stroke, I had lunch while sitting in a chair.

Shortly after, my occupational therapist returned—this time with a walking stick. She was pleased to see me eating in my chair and said that once I finished my meal, we could go for a short walk. She sat on my bed, waiting for me to finish eating, then gave me another ten minutes to let my food settle. Then, we set off.

She demonstrated how to use the walking stick, and I followed her lead as we walked down a long corridor—from one end of the building to the other. When we returned, she joked that I would have no trouble sleeping that night. I commented that I couldn't even remember the last time I had walked such a long distance since my stroke. Much to my delight, she said that her team would be happy to do this with me once a week. We agreed to make it a weekly session every Monday afternoon. From that day on, it truly felt like I was being prepared for rehabilitation.

PREPARATION FOR REHABILITATION

One of the nurses, who usually wiped me with a towel and warm water in bed every morning, came to me one evening before going home. She said she had been considering my request to have a male nurse take me to the shower room for a proper wash. She wanted me to ask my daughters to bring a sponge from home during their next visit because she had spoken to my caseworker, and they had agreed to team up to help me with the shower. I texted one of my daughters and got a sponge from home the following morning. It seemed a turning point for me in that hospital because they have a shower chair, which is pretty much like a wheelchair but made with plastic rather than leather upholstery.

One nurse would push me into the shower room, and on one occasion, my occupational therapist came in with us and demonstrated how to fix the shower so I could sit down to complete the process all by myself. After doing that with the nurses a few times, it became a routine for us and the two nurses would come to me by mid-morning and take me to have my shower. It felt like I had found two guardian angels, and we lived happily ever after until I got into more trouble with the so-called deputy ward manager again.

It kicked off when he came to my bedside to find me chatting with my two guardian angels. He walked over and joined our conversation, and I told the two nurses that this man refused to help me because he thought I was a risk of falling down and then that I found his behaviour unprofessional. That sort of wilful neglect would be gross misconduct in any corporate environment. He got angry and shouted at me, saying that if I ever went and mentioned his name anywhere, I would see what he would do to me. Although I regarded that as a threat, decided not to give him an audience, and ignored him completely, the female nurse laughed and said jokingly, "Do not let him talk to you like that". I smiled and pretended I did not hear what she said because an inner voice spoke to me, saying that I neither came to fix a broken hospital nor to make people upset, plus there was no point in adding fuel to the fire and risk escalating that matter any further.

My occupational therapist spoke to the two guardian angel nurses. Eventually, they began to push me onto the toilet for me to empty my bowels every morning as part of my shower process. By then, I could hold on to the grab rail next to the toilet if the nurses positioned me close enough, so I transferred onto the toilet by myself and only needed help to get cleaned and to come off when I finished using the toilet. The cleaning process would always end with my shower, and I would be taken back into the ward to get help to change into clean clothes and get ready for the day.

One morning, after my shower, my occupational therapist told me that I would need to be assessed by several rehabilitation units they were hoping to transfer me to. However, due to COVID restrictions, the assessments must be done virtually. The dates had already been set, so it was just a matter of informing me to prepare myself. I had two assessments that week and one more the following week, after which I was told I might be transferred the following week.

Next week, two ambulance crew members came into the ward with a wheelchair accompanied by my occupational therapist. My heart skipped a beat when she brought them to my bedside and spilt the beans immediately without mincing words. She told me to get my stuff ready because I was being transferred to a rehabilitation unit. I said my goodbyes very quickly and sat in the wheelchair. The ambulance crew members who had started to make their way out of the ward whisked me into the lift and downstairs into the car park. I thanked my occupational therapist and told her to say a special thank you to my two guardian angels. I followed the ambulance crew out of the ward into the lift, thinking that it was a good thing I wore my oversized jumper because it was not a warm day despite the bright spring sunshine.

LIVING WITH BRAIN INJURY - LIFE IN THE NEW NORMAL - I

The brain injury that I suffered utterly altered my life from a non-disabled independent person to a very ill person with limbs on one half of my body, which had been rendered inactive by the stroke and so cannot move without help from the opposite limb from the other side of my body; unfortunately, this has made me dependent on other people for help with basic tasks which require the use of both hands like wearing my shoes and my clothes.

There was hardly any need for me to wear my shoes during the days I was on admission at Hospital One because I was too weak to walk around the ward, so most of my time was spent in bed, and it was pretty much the same for the other patients. The nurses and therapists would help us wear our hospital pyjamas before bed at night.

My entire experience with the brain injury I suffered since the stroke has been challenging, but doing some research about the illness and condition has broadened my understanding. I visited the websites of the stroke association and affiliated organisations. I was able to read several stories of other patients and stroke survivors. I discovered that help was readily available from several organisations like the Queen Elizabeth Foundation for disabled people and other charities like the Shoreditch Trust and MIND.

I also discovered that these organisations provide the same support but slightly different ways to suit various needs. However, that was not surprising because brain injury affects everybody differently., I even applied for a driving assessment because I sent my driving license back to the DVLA after completing a medical questionnaire they sent me. Still, it was very clear that I applied for the driving assessment too early, and it made sense for me to recover more before applying again. So I shifted my focus to more physiotherapy sessions to improve my mobility because, at that moment, I still found it a little bit difficult to get in and out of cars, and that was one of the main concerns because in the event of an emergency if I needed to get out of the vehicle swiftly that would pose a problem. As a result, I decided to take a long break from driving because I was currently on retirement for medical reasons, so I need to move away from that self-denial mode and accept that my life has changed for the short and medium term. After meticulous consideration, I realised that I needed to become very serious about adjusting my life accordingly to make as much recovery as possible.

My social worker and occupational therapist from Hospital Three provided details of a social worker and the community therapist team from my local authority. I contacted them soon after arriving home after my final discharge from Hospital Three, and a small team of community therapists came to me shortly after. They recommended modifications to be made to our home. For example, they arranged for a bannister on our staircase to facilitate my walking up and down the stairs and make life easier for me.

They also prescribed suitable furniture, including a perching stool which I can sit on to look outside our home through my bedroom window to get a clear view of our road, and this provided me with a perfect way of getting out of bed and sitting behind my bedroom window to view our neighbourhood without the need to come outside the house. I also sat on the perching stool in front of my bathroom sink to brush my teeth every morning.

Some of the other items provided for me by the therapist included a walking stick and a shower chair because it was impossible for me to access my bath to bathe.

The therapists visited me a few times to show my family how to bring me downstairs. The idea was that my family members would show the social carers how to take me downstairs. Therefore, I could go downstairs with assistance from one member of my household, which made it possible for me to have some of my meals downstairs rather than in the bedroom. The therapists also showed us how to use the shower chair to assist me in bathing and provided me with the details of a company which would be responsible for the regular maintenance of my wheelchair.

After providing me with assistance, including speech and language therapy sessions for a few weeks, I was discharged by the community therapists, and all my help and support became the responsibility of my family and my social care provider,

The social care providing company sent someone to carry out an assessment. Still, when she saw the process of taking me downstairs, she said their staff would not be allowed to help me go downstairs because it was unsafe for them to assist me when we were simultaneously on the staircase. Still, it became clear that they were passing the buck between themselves and the community therapists. Hence, the only way for me to go downstairs was with my family members, who became unpaid carers and were always willing to help and support me if they could. However, I do get a feeling and worry that they are getting overwhelmed because of the help and support that they have to provide for me daily. However, it remains my prayer that God Himself would give me complete healing and restore mobility to me entirely to provide them with relief from the overwhelming task that they are doing by helping me and support daily.

Before they discharged me, the community therapists suggested that I get help installing a stair lift to help me come downstairs regularly without assistance. However, they agreed with me that my stairway was very narrow, so it was decided that an installation engineer needed to go and have a look and take measurements for us to find the way forward, but it turned out that there was a long waiting list so I have to wait for the installation to be completed. I am still waiting for that to happen. They also said that climbing up and down the stairs was an excellent exercise for me. However, I must say that climbing downstairs with assistance from one person and climbing upstairs under supervision is a fantastic way to exercise my weak limbs.

I get invitations from the therapist team at Hospital One to come for monthly reviews. They have been beneficial in monitoring my progress and ensuring that everything is going as expected, and this monthly review is still an ongoing process. In the long term, my only option for going up and down the stairs at home is to pursue the installation of a stair lift and see how the waiting list situation unfolds. The conversation comes up every time I go to Hospital One for the monthly review, and I hope that something will be done about installing the stair lift. However, the outcome remains to be seen, so I guess I would have to continue asking my doctor to make referrals to the community therapist team and the social prescribers in my local authority until I get any information about when the installation would be carried out.

During my last review session, I explained that coming upstairs is becoming much more manageable and that I am improving with time. I told them I tried to come up with supervision rather than assistance, and therapists made a perfect point and suggested that the lift could help me come downstairs by myself. For me to climb back upstairs as often as I want to exercise my limbs, it goes without saying that coming downstairs with assistance has become a great form of exercise. That's what I'm doing at the moment. However, it would be even better if a stair lift were installed, as I could complete both the descent and ascent independently. This would be a significant step toward regaining my independence. Additionally, I could move freely between floors whenever I wanted, rather than waiting for assistance, as I have to now.

I also visited Hospital Three for Botox injections into my left limbs, which were affected by the stroke. It must be mentioned that Hospital One also provided what they called "Patient Initiated Follow-Up Appointments", another handy way to iron out any issues that arise or are still outstanding. Crucially, this helps to prevent that feeling of being lost in the maze. Hospital Two had been completely missing in action as far as any follow-up with my recovery was concerned. Still, sometimes no news was good news, so I would find out from my doctor because the staff at Hospital One asked me during one of my review visits if I did get any invitations from Hospital Two regarding follow up since my final discharge. I said no but did not ask if they were supposed to provide me with any follow-up or some help to check or monitor my progress.

I also have to say that I continue to receive invitations from the therapists at Hospital One for a monthly review. They constantly assess me and have discussions to ensure I am making the expected progress. They also make recommendations to my doctor and referrals to my community therapist team and social prescribers in my local authority if needed. Unfortunately, most of these recommendations fail to materialise due to waiting lists and/or lack of funding.

LIVING WITH BRAIN INJURY - MANAGING FATIGUE

I found sleeping very difficult at night mainly, and my staying in bed virtually all day was not helpful as well because I did not have the opportunity to burn off energy, even though I had always been a very active person before suffering the stroke and not used to staying in bed for long periods. As a result, I ended up being tired from spending too much time in bed and over time, this began to cause fatigue, which in turn began to affect my night sleep. It felt like I was trapped in a vicious cycle of sleeplessness and fatigue because I was waking up in the mornings feeling tired and exhausted.

My night sleep improved gradually as the days went by, and I began to walk indoors as much as possible as I continued to adapt to life after discharge from the hospital. I started walking pretty soon after waking up; I walked into the bathroom to use the toilet, although I did require assistance from at least one person to come off when I had finished my business. My wife does that for me every morning before going to work.

I walked to the bathroom daily to brush my teeth by sitting on a perching stool in front of the sink. Another contribution to my lack of sleep was that everything I did was in bed. I was getting assistance from my wife to get an accurate shower using the shower chair provided by the community therapist. I gradually got the routine of getting a shower three times a week. Still, it wasn't easy for my wife and I to consider having a shower more than once a day, so we decided to stick to the three days and added Saturday as well because she does not work on Saturday. Other than that, we only bothered when I had to go outside for a hospital appointment or some other reason.

I could walk into the bathroom and sit on my perching stool just a few days into my recovery. Since there weren't many options for the nurses, it wasn't about damage limitation but taking things one day at a time.

I began having conversations and making friends, and life became a bit more interesting once more. Occasionally, when my family came to visit, the nurses would help me to transfer into my wheelchair and pushed out of the ward to sit outside the hospital entrance with them in the hospital's main reception area. We all used to enjoy those moments because it felt much better than just watching me lie in bed for the entire duration of their visit. It was also an opportunity for us to have quality time together as a family. Personally, it was also an opportunity to spend some time out of bed and outside the hospital ward.

I quickly learned that if walking was possible, getting out of the ward, even for short periods, helped me burn off some energy. This gave me quality sleep at night to replenish that energy, which was key to resolving my fatigue issue. Without even realising it, I began getting quality, sound sleep, which helped me wake up in the mornings with a fresh feeling of being restored and rested, enabling me to work even harder in the gym.

As time went on, I realised that my night sleep greatly improved on days that I had exercise sessions with the therapist, and for patients still in the hospital, the therapists would always be glad to help if they were asked for help with the exercise in any shape or form.

Depending on the patient's stage, their recovery-for example, at the very early stages, it was not always possible to do any meaningful exercise, although even stretches and massaging could be beneficial and were better than nothing.

Simply lying in bed for extended periods during recovery wasn't an option for me. Instead, I used my static bike to exercise my limbs or walked up and down the gym's stairs if the hospital had that facility. Whatever the situation, patients should take advantage of the healthcare professionals around them for supervised walking or light exercise, which can contribute to better sleep at night.

I was pretty sure the therapists would always be happy to help any patient willing to take the initiative to become more active rather than spending long periods in bed. For me, being active helped prevent the fatigue that can sometimes come with lying around, allowing me to get quality sleep and wake up feeling rested. As for other patients still admitted, simple activities like walking around the ward with supervision from healthcare professionals or making regular trips to the bathroom to brush their teeth or use the toilet could be small but helpful steps toward long-term recovery. It's all about those little actions that, over time, make a big difference.

CHAPTER 3
TRIALS AND TRIUMPHS

One day, my consultant, who informed me that I would soon be transferred to a hospital closer to my residence and referred me to Hospital Two, explained that, due to my continued progress and positive response to treatment, I would be going for rehabilitation shortly. While this should have been good news, I was deeply disappointed. Hospital Two had a terrible reputation, and I dreaded being sent there. Nonetheless, at the beginning of the following week, I was once again transported by ambulance to this new facility.

To my relief, it was indeed more manageable for my family to visit, and they took full advantage of this, coming far more frequently than before. Even better, my health improved significantly. I started sitting up in a chair beside my bed and was able to transfer into my wheelchair without assistance. However, I still spent most of my days in bed, and my routine remained essentially unchanged.

One evening, I asked a nurse—introduced to me as my caseworker—to provide me with a commode, a wheelchair-like toilet seat that could be positioned over a regular toilet. To my horror, the nurse coldly refused, stating that such assistance was not provided in the evening. His only task would have been to push me onto the toilet seat, yet he chose to walk away instead.

This refusal was callous, given that one of the evening medications I received was a laxative. Denying me access to a toilet after administering such medication meant that any discomfort I experienced overnight would become the responsibility of the night staff. That night, I lay awake in terrible pain, my belly aching intensely. In desperation, I pressed the call button, and a night shift nurse finally brought me the commode, allowing me some relief before I managed to get a little sleep.

The following day, my consultant arrived and, as usual, opened his laptop. He asked me what had happened between 1 a.m. and 3:30 a.m. because the readings from my heart monitor showed irregular activity. Knowing how meticulous he was, I told him the truth—that I had been in severe pain because I couldn't access the toilet. He advised me always to call the nurses, as that was their job. I agreed outwardly, but internally, I knew that I was dealing with a flawed system that I had no power to fix. Later, I asked a day nurse why they administered laxatives at night but refused to help patients use the toilet. She simply laughed and said, "Don't let them treat you like that!"—a response that stunned me but also revealed how deeply embedded these issues were.

Unfortunately, I began to experience hostility from some of the nursing staff at Hospital Two. When the lead consultant asked for my feedback, I spoke candidly about the lack of management and accountability. I pointed out how nurses would often disappear from the stroke ward precisely when patients needed assistance the most. When I inquired about this, I was told they were on break— whenever they chose—because they were not paid for their breaks. I was shocked, as I had assumed employment laws required paid breaks after a certain number of working hours.

I also noticed a disturbing lack of trade union presence, which could have addressed many of these systemic issues. My standing among the nurses worsened when I challenged one for speaking rudely to an elderly patient. Another nurse retaliated by claiming that many NHS patients were misdiagnosed because they displayed attitudes like mine. This particular nurse, I later discovered, was the deputy ward manager.

Things escalated further when he falsely labelled me as a fall risk, leading the nurses to avoid me. One morning, as he passed my bed, I asked for help repositioning myself, but he shouted that he wouldn't touch me because he'd be blamed if I fell. He walked off, even after I pointed out the consultant's note on my bedside indicating I required assistance. When I accused him of neglect, he became furious and questioned whether I was an NHS investigator or a patient. He then threatened me, warning that if I ever mentioned his name, I would "see what he would do to me". I chose to ignore the threat, not wanting to escalate the situation further.

Despite these challenges, I remained committed to my therapy. The sessions were not too intense, as I was still in the early stages of recovery, but they marked a turning point for me. The therapists started taking me out of bed for walks around the ward with the aid of walking support. They also began assisting me with toilet visits, demonstrating to the nurses that I could transfer from my wheelchair to the toilet independently. This encouraged some of the nurses to be more supportive. One male nurse, in particular, stood out—he disregarded the negative rumours about me and began helping me regularly. His kindness meant the world to me. He even took the time to say goodbye at the end of his shifts and let me know what time he would return the following day to assist with my shower.

Another nurse also touched my heart when she noticed that I had potential but was spending too much time in bed. With the weather improving, she offered to take me outside for fresh air. I eagerly accepted, and she regularly wheeled me to the hospital car park. These small acts of compassion completely transformed my perception of Hospital Two.

One evening, as the nurses ended their shift, they wrote in the handover notes that I was depressed. The following morning, a doctor, puzzled by this note, visited me. He found me in high spirits, chatting and joking with fellow patients. He admitted that he had initially considered prescribing antidepressants but was glad he had checked on me first. When I later inquired which nurse had made the false report, he said it was impossible to determine. This deeply unsettled me—it illustrated how easily patients could be misdiagnosed and how little accountability existed within the system.

As my time at Hospital Two neared its end, I was assessed for transfer to a rehabilitation unit. My consultant informed me that I could be transferred within a week, and I prepared myself for this next step. When the day arrived, two ambulance crew members arrived at my bedside, and my therapist helped me gather my belongings. After saying my goodbyes, I was on my way to Hospital Three.

Upon arrival, I was placed in a private side ward due to ongoing COVID-19 restrictions. The nurses welcomed me warmly, showed me the call bell, and reassured me that I could reach out if I needed anything. My wife soon arrived, beaming with joy at my improved state. Over the next few days, I met with my new consultant and occupational therapist, who explained that the focus in the rehabilitation unit was on preparing patients for independent living. Unlike a standard hospital setting, the emphasis was on regaining self-sufficiency.

Patients followed a structured schedule that included therapy sessions in the gym, speech and language therapy, and occupational training. Meals were served in a designated dining area, and patients were encouraged to eat there instead of in their rooms. In my first week, a nurse would wheel me to the dining hall, but the goal was for me to walk there independently over time. The unit also had a large gym, where each patient had scheduled time slots for rehabilitation exercises.

Prior to my discharge, the therapists and I set a personal challenge: I would leave the hospital walking with my stick rather than in a wheelchair. It was an ambitious yet achievable goal, as I had already begun taking steps with assistance. When my discharge day arrived, I was filled with joy as I walked into my daughter's car in the hospital parking lot, a moment of triumph I will never forget.

Despite the hardships I endured across three different hospitals, my journey brought me even closer to God. The challenges tested my faith, but they also strengthened it, and for that, I am grateful. Looking back, I can see that even in my darkest moments, there were blessings hidden in the struggle.

MY REHABILITATION JOURNEY: TRANSFER TO HOSPITAL THREE AND MANAGING FATIGUE AFTER BRAIN INJURY

A few prospective rehabilitation units assessed me for a possible transfer, though all assessments were conducted virtually due to COVID-19 restrictions. My consultant informed me after one such evaluation that I could be transferred within a week, so I began preparing myself for the move. This was expected to be my final hospital admission since, if everything went well in the rehabilitation unit, I would be discharged directly from there to go home.

One afternoon, I saw two ambulance crew members on the ward. They were brought to my bedside by one of the therapists, who told me to gather my belongings as I was being transferred to another hospital. I bid farewell and expressed my gratitude to the nurses and fellow patients before leaving. Within minutes, we were on our way, and we arrived at Hospital Three in the late afternoon, approaching early evening.

Upon arrival, I was taken to a minor side ward with no other patients, apparently due to COVID regulations still being in place. The room had its own sink and a small TV.

Several nurses came in to introduce themselves, which made me feel welcomed. They showed me a bell and instructed me to press it if I needed anything at all. I settled in quickly, and my wife arrived soon after I finished my dinner. She was overjoyed to see me so happy.

I also had visits from the occupational therapist and my new consultant, who walked me through the basics of how rehabilitation care differs from regular hospital care. One notable difference was the emphasis on preparing patients for life outside the hospital, with an expectation for patients to do as much as they possibly could for themselves—especially with basic daily tasks like brushing their teeth. Each patient followed a structured schedule, ensuring clear routines and detailed plans for therapy and other sessions. Physiotherapy sessions took place in the gym with the occupational therapist, while speech and language therapy sessions were conducted in a much smaller seminar room.

After two weeks, I was moved to the central ward. Meals were served in a designated dining area, and patients were encouraged to eat there. Whether attending occupational therapy in the gym or speech and language therapy in a seminar room, one remarkable difference was the structured daily program. It detailed my daily activities, and meals were served twice daily in a separate dining area with tables and chairs. For the first week, my assigned nurse pushed me to the dining area for meals, but over time, I was expected to walk there myself using my walking aids and return to my ward afterwards. The nurses were always available to administer my medication by the time we finished our meals. The hospital had a large gym with various equipment, and each patient had scheduled time slots on specific days for their therapy sessions.

I was provided with a chair beside my bed, a wheelchair, and a walking stick. I spent a lot of time in bed, just like I did in the previous two hospitals. However, I regularly rang the bell for nurses to help me transfer into my wheelchair or the chair beside my bed, preventing me from lying in bed all day. Sometimes, I sat in my wheelchair and watched television instead. Each evening, I checked my schedule and prepared myself for the next day's activities. There were two mornings each week when therapists assisted me in the bathroom for a shower. Additionally, every Wednesday, I was asked to wear my own clothes instead of hospital attire because that was the day allocated for therapists and nurses to take me out of the ward to other parts of the hospital.

Before my discharge from Hospital Three, the therapist and I set a mutual challenge for myself: to leave the hospital walking with my stick rather than in a wheelchair, as I had arrived. Since I was already capable of doing this, I gladly accepted the challenge. On the day of my discharge, I was overjoyed to walk to my daughter's car in the hospital parking lot.

The harrowing experience of being admitted to three different hospitals and the complete transformation of my life has drawn me even closer to God. Looking back, I am grateful that, despite the challenges brought by the stroke I suffered, I can see at least one positive outcome from it all.

LIVING WITH BRAIN INJURY – LIFE IN THE NEW NORMAL - II

After spending seven to eight months in three different hospitals, I was finally discharged and transitioned to the community therapist team in my borough. The occupational therapist and social worker from the last hospital provided me with details of the community therapy team and a social worker. Upon contacting them, they responded swiftly, and soon after, the therapists visited me. It was a small team consisting of a technician, an occupational therapist, and a speech and language therapist.

The technician assessed the equipment needed to make my daily life more manageable. Within days, a bannister was installed on my staircase for support, and I was given a high-rise chair for my sitting room, making it easier to get up without assistance. The occupational therapist provided me with a schedule for my speech and language therapy sessions and coordinated my social care provision. They arranged for an assessor from the adult social care team of the local authority to conduct a risk assessment. The care provider then finalised arrangements, including the frequency and timing of social carers' visits. A key safe was installed to ensure easy access for carers and healthcare workers, which was arranged by the technician and set up within a few days.

Diet

A balanced diet is crucial for anyone recovering from a brain injury. While hospital meals are typically healthy, dietary habits often decline post-discharge. Many stroke survivors end up consuming unhealthy food due to convenience or affordability, which can reverse the progress made in the hospital.

Through my research, I've realised that moving away from ultra-processed foods is a significant step toward recovery. However, this can be difficult for patients without family support to help with meal preparation. A good rule of thumb is to avoid excessive carbohydrates and focus on fibre-rich foods, mainly fruits and vegetables, which aid digestion and overall well-being. Diet, combined with regular exercise, plays a crucial role in rehabilitation, but for many recovering patients, access to both can be challenging.

One of my most memorable moments during rehabilitation was the day I decided to walk around the hospital. With the encouragement of my occupational therapist, I grabbed my walking stick and ventured through the ward, supported by my therapist, who followed closely with a wheelchair. Other patients and staff cheered me on as I made my way outside to the car park. That evening, the ward manager praised my determination, especially considering the severity of my stroke. The next day, I noticed a significant reduction in my medication, and upon inquiring, the nurse informed me that my physical activity had contributed to the change.

Managing Fatigue

Fatigue has been one of the biggest challenges in my new normal. Following my therapy sessions, I often sleep deeply and wake up feeling drained. Fortunately, I am on medical retirement, so I don't have to worry about returning to work. Public transportation has also become difficult, but my social worker and occupational therapist arranged a London taxi card for me. Although I booked in advance, getting into the taxi remains a challenge due to a big step that I struggled to climb without assistance. The journey itself can be rough due to speed ramps, but I have learned to manage.

My family takes care of household shopping and other tasks I previously handled. I voluntarily surrendered my driving license to the DVLA and have no immediate plans to resume driving. Instead, I focus on maintaining a healthy lifestyle, which includes a nutritious diet and regular exercise. Brisk walking in my local park is part of my routine, though it's not always possible. In such cases, I do simple stretching exercises at home using my strong arm to support and strengthen my weaker arm. Even small movements are better than none, as they prevent stiffness and promote circulation.

LIFE AFTER RECOVERING FROM BRAIN INJURY

One key piece of advice from healthcare professionals has been to avoid overthinking. While it's difficult not to dwell on my condition, I try to focus on what I can control rather than worrying about things beyond my power. Writing this book has been a way to distract me from my worries, primarily since I am not used to being at home all day without work. However, I consider myself fortunate to have access to technology, allowing me to watch live TV and other content from the comfort of my bed when I feel too tired to go downstairs.

During one of my hospital visits, the community therapists offered to install a stair lift in my home to help me move between floors. I declined the offer because walking up and down the stairs has become an essential exercise for me. Additionally, my narrow staircase would have made a stair lift inconvenient for my family. As a result, I now limit most of my indoor walking to the first floor of my house.

Leaving the house is another challenge, as I require assistance to step outside. Because of this, I only go out when necessary, such as for hospital appointments. Eventually, I hired a private therapist to accompany me on walks around my neighbourhood and local park, though brisk walking remains a long-term goal. Fatigue is another barrier, requiring someone to push my wheelchair when I need to rest.

Over time, it has become evident that my family is becoming overwhelmed with their caregiving responsibilities. My occupational therapist suggested that I be referred to a social worker who could arrange a personal assistant for me. However, the waiting period for such services is long, and I have no way of knowing whether progress is being made. As a last resort, I reached out to my doctor's office, only to be told by their social prescriber that I must wait indefinitely. I can only hope that help eventually comes.

Despite these challenges, I remain optimistic about my recovery. I believe that in time, I will be able to work again, perhaps in a hybrid job that allows me to work from home. For now, I take things one day at a time—resting when I need to, exercising as much as possible, and hoping for continued progress. As the weather improves, I look forward to walking outside more frequently, with the support of my family or therapist. Until then, I remind myself that every small step forward is a victory and a testament to my resilience.

Barriers

One of the personal barriers I have encountered is my inability to put on my shoes by myself. As a result, I am considering investing in footwear that I can easily slip on. However, the key requirement is that the footwear must provide stability, so I tend to avoid Crocs, sliders, and other typical easy-to-wear shoes for safety reasons, as my safety remains my utmost priority. The difficulty in finding suitable footwear arises because it is very challenging for me to walk barefoot, even indoors. This was something my therapists strongly emphasised before my discharge from the hospital. I must admit that walking without shoes indoors is still a work in progress for me, but the sooner I overcome this barrier, the sooner I can grab my walking stick and move around my bedroom independently. This would also allow me to transition to wearing slippers or sliders without assistance—something I greatly look forward to in my journey to regain independence.

Positives

Generally speaking, adjusting to the new normal is different for every stroke survivor, which is hardly surprising, given that a stroke affects individuals in unique ways. Some patients take longer to recover than others, and some require more frequent medical attention. However, one universal truth for all stroke survivors is that the experience not only reshapes but also highlights the everyday activities we once took for granted. For instance, simple acts of helping one another within a family unit and working together harmoniously to provide support become essential, as the stroke survivor's limited ability to contribute may create a gap that needs to be filled to maintain a functional household. These changes necessitate adjustments and modifications to the so-called "new normal".

Although what I call "life in the new normal" has the potential to strengthen family bonds, it can also expose existing cracks, sometimes even leading to strained relationships. For some families, however, it serves as an opportunity to foster deeper connections, ultimately helping them navigate life's challenges together. One realisation I had early on was that many of the carers employed by my social care provider to support me have personal experiences with stroke-affected family members. Strangely, this underscores how a stroke can have far-reaching impacts—not just on the individual but on their loved ones as well.

The key takeaway for stroke survivors is to recognise that they are not alone. Seeking help from charities and voluntary organisations can provide the necessary support for both survivors and their families. I hope that any stroke survivor reading this article finds some reassurance in knowing that support is available and they do not have to face these challenges in isolation.

The New Normal

Technological innovations, combined with support from government and voluntary organisations, have made life significantly easier for stroke patients striving to regain aspects of their pre-stroke lives. These discussions should ideally take place during the final rehabilitation process before hospital discharge. I was fortunate to have therapists, social workers, and clinical psychologists address these matters before I even had to ask.

One significant aspect of my hospital experience was the adaptations made to assist me. For instance, a nurse took it upon himself to dismiss concerns about my fall risk and ensured I received a proper shower daily. This small act of kindness significantly improved my hospital stay, and my family was delighted when I requested sponges and soaps after sharing the good news. It reassured me that there were indeed hardworking and compassionate nurses in the hospital. Unfortunately, there were also individuals whose actions undermined the dedicated efforts of these few good professionals. A little scrutiny and accountability within the hospital system could go a long way in improving the overall patient experience and restoring faith in healthcare services.

In summary, living with a brain injury is highly subjective and depends on individual circumstances, as well as the level of support available from carers and healthcare professionals. I have witnessed survivors living in communal flats where long corridors with lifts at both ends make it much easier for them to access local shops and parks with minimal assistance.

It remains my hope that other brain injury survivors can reflect on my experiences and adapt them to their own situations, enabling them to transition to the new normal as smoothly as possible. Additionally, I hope healthcare professionals reading this piece gain insight into a patient's perspective, allowing them to refine their approach and enhance the quality of care they provide. Lastly, student therapists and trainee healthcare professionals may also find value in this article, offering them a real-world glimpse into the challenges faced by stroke survivors and the impact of compassionate care.

Living through the challenges of stroke recovery is undeniably tough, but it is also a journey of self-discovery, growth, and resilience. The barriers we face, whether physical, emotional, or psychological, can feel insurmountable at times, but with the proper support, resources, and mindset, recovery is not only possible but empowering. The journey to the new normal is different for everyone, but it's important to remember that it is not one we must walk alone. Family, friends, carers, and healthcare professionals all play pivotal roles in ensuring that stroke survivors are not just surviving but thriving.

Though the road ahead may seem daunting, the potential for stronger relationships, greater self-sufficiency, and a renewed sense of independence is within reach. Every small victory—whether it's taking a step on your own or putting on shoes without help—represents a significant milestone. It's these victories, along with the compassion and understanding of those around us, that will ultimately make the "new normal" a fulfilling and hopeful reality.

For stroke survivors reading this, remember that you are stronger than you may realise, and there is always support available. For healthcare professionals, please take this opportunity to view recovery through the eyes of your patients, as it will undoubtedly improve the care you provide. Together, we can create a world where every stroke survivor has the tools, support, and understanding they need to reclaim their life and their independence.

www.ingramcontent.com/pod-product-compliance
Lightning Source LLC
Chambersburg PA
CBHW071525210326
41597CB00018B/2895